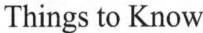

Things to Know

50 THINGS TO KNOW BOOK SERIES REVIEWS FROM READERS

I recently downloaded a couple of books from this series to read over the weekend thinking I would read just one or two. However, I so loved the books that I read all the six books I had downloaded in one go and ended up downloading a few more today. Written by different authors, the books offer practical advice on how you can perform or achieve certain goals in life, which in this case is how to have a better life.

The information is simple to digest and learn from, and is incredibly useful. There are also resources listed at the end of the book that you can use to get more information.

50 Things To Know To Have A Better Life: Self-Improvement Made Easy!

Author Dannii Cohen

This book is very helpful and provides simple tips on how to improve your everyday life. I found it to be useful in improving my overall attitude.

50 Things to Know For Your Mindfulness & Meditation Journey
Author Nina Edmondso

Quick read with 50 short and easy tips for what to think about before starting to homeschool.

50 Things to Know About Getting Started with Homeschool by Author Amanda Walton

I really enjoyed the voice of the narrator, she speaks in a soothing tone. The book is a really great reminder of things we might have known we could do during stressful times, but forgot over the years.

Author Harmony Hawaii

There is so much waste in our society today. Everyone should be forced to read this book. I know I am passing it on to my family.

50 Things to Know to Downsize Your Life: How To Downsize, Organize, And Get Back to Basics

Author Lisa Rusczyk Ed. D.

Great book to get you motivated and understand why you may be losing motivation. Great for that person who wants to start getting healthy, or just for you when you need motivation while having an established workout routine.

50 Things To Know To Stick With A Workout: Motivational Tips To Start The New You Today

Author Sarah Hughes

THINGS TO KNOW ABOUT PARENTING A PEDIATRIC ~~CANCER~~ SURVIVOR

Our Story of Battling the Beast

Valerie Kline

Things to Know About Parenting a Pediatric Cancer Survivor Copyright © 2021 by CZYK Publishing LLC. All Rights Reserved.

All rights reserved. No part of this book may be reproduced in any form or by any electronic or mechanical means including information storage and retrieval systems, without permission in writing from the author. The only exception is by a reviewer, who may quote short excerpts in a review.

The statements in this book are of the authors and may not be the views of CZYK Publishing or 50 Things to Know.

Cover designed by: Ivana Stamenkovic
Cover Image: https://pixabay.com/photos/life-beauty-scene-achieve-862985/

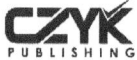

CZYK Publishing Since 2011.
CZYKPublishing.com
50 Things to Know

Lock Haven, PA
All rights reserved.
ISBN: 9798492435271

THINGS TO KNOW ABOUT PARENTING A PEDIATRIC ~~CANCER~~ SURVIVOR

BOOK DESCRIPTION

What would you do if your child was diagnosed with cancer? Who would you reach out to? How would you and your family survive?

If you want to know the answer to any of these questions, then this book is for you.

Things to Know About Parenting a Pediatric Cancer Survivor: Our Story of Battling the Beast, by Valerie Kline, offers an insight to pediatric cancer treatment that comes from personal experience. Most books on the topic tell you the facts and statistics, or ask for donations. Although there's nothing wrong with that, this book offers an insider's story combined with knowledge from research and experts.

In these pages you'll bear witness to the strength and courage, weakness and hopelessness that comes with parenting a pediatric cancer survivor. This book can help you navigate the wily road of cancer treatment and recovery.

By the time you finish this book, you will know how to learn from and let go of the worst experience a parent can live through. You will be warned of the overwhelming challenges - physical, mental, and emotional. You will understand the resources available to you and why to ask for help. There will be facts and terminology used to explain the various treatments available for the many types and stages of cancer. There will be stories that break your heart and stories that offer hope. Whether you are a parent, or know a parent, grab YOUR copy today. You'll be glad you did.

TABLE OF CONTENTS

50 Things to Know
Book Series
Reviews from Readers
BOOK DESCRIPTION
TABLE OF CONTENTS
DEDICATION
ABOUT THE AUTHOR
INTRODUCTION
LIFE BEFORE CANCER
DIAGNOSIS
TREATMENT
RESOURCES
MORE TREATMENT
OUR LIFE CURRENTLY
Other Helpful Resources
50 Things to Know

Things to Know

DEDICATION

In honor of all the angel cancer kids who fought hard and found peace.

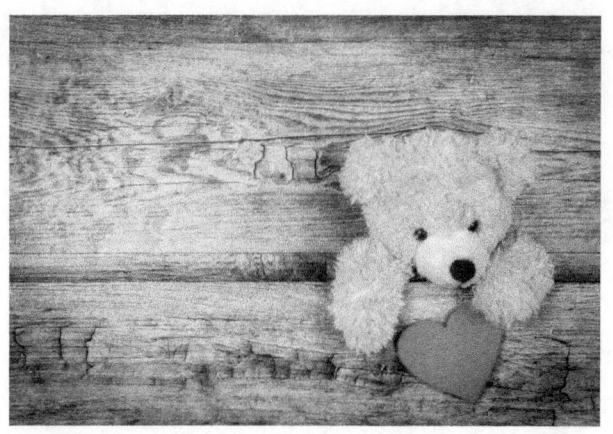

Things to Know

ABOUT THE AUTHOR

I was born in Rockford, Illinois, and grew up in Geneseo, Illinois, a small town almost in Iowa. I grew up on a farm and know the value of hard-work, community, and passion. After high school, I attended Western Illinois University, where I earned both my undergraduate and Graduate degree in English. I also played volleyball and participated in a number of clubs and activities while in college. After college, I moved back to her hometown and eventually got married to my college beau. He taught physical education and I taught high school and college English for over a decade, caring for multiple pets, raising two daughters, and overcoming whatever obstacles life threw at us.

When our youngest daughter was diagnosed with cancer at the age of thirteen months, our world stopped. After two grueling years of family separation because of chemotherapy and radiation treatments, life began to resume its normal pace. Our daughter is currently free of treatment and goes in periodically for maintenance scans and check-ups. She is one of the lucky survivors and has inspired this book. #NoOneFightsAlone

During these years, I used my writing as an outlet for expression and therapy. After my daughter's treatment, I resumed teaching, but just did not have the heart for it. Instead of pouring myself into other people's children, I needed to focus my time and energy on my own. I gave up teaching, although education is still a passion of mine, and now keep a shop in a little store in my hometown while I work on my novels and writing projects.

I attend soccer, softball, and volleyball practices for my eleven-year-old, Penny, and kindergarten programs and parties for my healthy, active five-year-old, Evelyn. My parents and extended family remain an important part of my life, even though my younger brother moved to Australia nearly seven years ago. I plan to visit to celebrate finishing my Three Brothers Heritage Trilogy. There are several mottos I live by, depending on what I need during the day: "Unless someone like you cares a whole awful lot, nothing's going to get better. It's not," from Doctor Suess's the Lorax, or "And though she be but little, she is fierce," from Shakespeare.

Things to Know

You can find me here:

Facebook - The Works of Valerie Jean

Instagram - valerie_jean83

Twitter - valkline83

Blog - My-romantic.com

INTRODUCTION

> *"We don't know how strong we are until being strong is the only choice we have."*

While writing this, I could hardly make it through a blurb or paragraph without breaking down crying. It didn't make me feel strong. Getting it out has been part nightmare, and part therapy. However, I had to get it out there. For so many reasons beyond just my own mental health.

> *"Some people never meet their hero. I gave birth to mine."*

My child was forced to be a hero too soon, as are too many others. Many people don't realize the trauma and sacrifice and loss that goes into cancer treatment, even if you do beat the disease. Her developmental years were spent in and out of hospitals, being poisoned and primed to fight the disease killing her from the inside out. There are so many odds stacked against childhood cancer patients. And the world needs to start realizing that what we're doing is not enough. Making a profit off of cancer medicines shouldn't even be on the radar of priorities. Researching, tracking, studying, experimenting, and funding for childhood cancer patients and treatments needs to start taking priority. Too many children are getting diagnosed with too many diseases requiring too many medicines that aren't being created. So writing this became necessary to bring awareness to others.

    A nurse clinician, Suzanne Horn, from British Columbia Children's Hospital Foundation described the unfairness of it all extremely well:

Things to Know

*"They ride tricycles in the hallway,
not in the park.
They know the names of their chemos
instead of their classmates.
Their central lines have names.
Nurses and doctors are their new family.
They think hair is overrated.
Their laughter can make a grown person cry.
If you've ever seen a kid fight cancer,
it will change your life."*

Things to Know

LIFE BEFORE CANCER

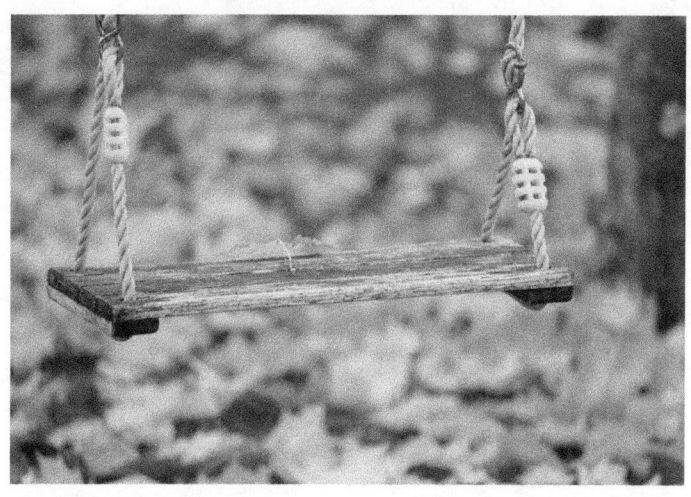

Things to Know

I was pushing my toddler, Evelyn Rose, in her swing in the backyard on a Friday in March of 2017 when I first listened to the nurse's voicemail. According to the lab results from her twelve month wellness check, she had low iron. They were going to send us to Peoria next week for some tests with a specific hematologist and oncologist. They warned us that her counts were so low that if she hit her head or got a scratch, we needed to watch for excessive bleeding. We had no idea she was at such a high risk of serious injury. Evelyn had been an active, healthy child since she was born. She was coordinated, agile, and hit all of her developmental markers right on time. She woke up with the sun and went to bed after it set most days. Keeping her safe and inactive all weekend long was a task in itself. Little did we know that task would take over our lives for the next two years.

Looking back on that weekend, it was the last full weekend we'd be at home together as a family for the next two years. I'm not sure what we did. We may have attended a sporting event for our older daughter, Penelope. We may have just stayed at home and caught up around the house. I wish I would have paid more attention to the daily details. Never take for granted the time you get at home with family. Penny would be single-parented, or living with Grandma and Grandpa, or staying with friends throughout the next two years. When Ian or I were home, we were shells of parents to her. I missed her carefree, loving personality and watching her athletic talents in soccer and softball. My parents were an ever-present ghost in my life, helping and haunting at the same time. They wanted to make life easier, but yearned for understanding about how our priorities in life had changed. They cleaned our house, took care of our pets, and watched Penelope for us. Our friends tried to be understanding and supportive, but couldn't comprehend the challenges or misery. Where I had once been an optimistic, positive influence in a room, I could hardly hold it together around people anymore. I came to resent people for living a normal life. We slowly disappeared from any and all social circles in order to survive.

Taking Evelyn to Peoria for that first appointment, we had little to no warning that she was about to be tested, treated, and tormented for the developmental years of her life. We got lost on the way there, causing us to stress and fight more than normal. The address our GPS pulled up wasn't the accurate address anymore because medical practices are always changing and relocating. We came to learn this was normal in the medical community, which often caused confusion and frustration. Our GPS led us through a run-down, somewhat scary-looking area of Peoria. We finally found the right building by calling someone and having them give directions, then actually stopping and asking someone else for better directions. The appointment ended up being on the other side of town from where we were, which meant we were also late, only adding to our stress.

This was our first experience with the complicated medical system of hospitals, referrals, and specialists. Up until this, we'd had easy wellness checks with Penny. My husband and I hadn't been to a doctor for more than a physical in over ten years. It had always been a matter of visiting the doctor, submitting an insurance claim, and having it paid for. From here on out, it was a matter of organizing and balancing funds and shifting money to make life work. Insurance is a cruel system in the United States. How people view it as okay to profit off of other people's suffering is beyond me.

St. Jude's Children's Hospital is a lifesaver. Without their financial and emotional assistance, as well as medical research and treatment guidance, we may not have saved her. I know there are other hospitals and research foundations that offer high-quality treatment options, and I commend these as well. Children's Oncology Group (COG), M.D. Anderson Cancer Center, Dana-Farber Cancer Institute, Memorial Sloan Kettering Cancer Center, and Pediatric Brain Tumor Consortium are just some of the organizations and institutes that provide treatment and research on childhood cancer.

Walking into the small clinic in Peoria, Illinois, we had no idea how our life was going to change. I realize now that the nurses and doctors probably already knew what was coming. The nurse came in and did all of the regular paperwork, and asked all of the usual questions, then referred to the doctor. He took one quick look at Evelyn's abdomen and sent us to St. Jude. By quick I mean he examined her for less than sixty seconds. There was a six centimeter tumor in her belly, which explained several abnormalities that had been going on.

She'd had several rounds of mysterious fevers, which the doctors had given her antibiotics for. She also had bruises under her eyes that would come and go. Laying her on her back for diaper changes had made her distraught. Not just upset like an active baby; crying like she was being tortured. She had a couple episodes of vomiting while she was swinging as well, which was extremely odd. She loved her

Things to Know

swing. Finding this out made us understand that prioritizing medical checks was imperative. Getting in to see a doctor regularly is important. Although it's easy to be scared, or say just tough it out, do not ignore warning signs that could be symptoms of larger problems.

Sending us to St. Jude's Clinic at OSF St. Francis, we were zombies. I know my husband was as lost and overwhelmed as I was. My parents were watching Penny during this one day trip that had suddenly turned into an overnight one. At that point, we had no idea how many nights we'd actually be staying. Hearing that your toddler is going in for surgery is one of the most difficult things you'll hear as a parent. She had to undergo biopsies and tests to determine the specific type of cancer and the staging of it. They had to warn us of all the possible side effects of anesthesia as well as the surgery. Her tumor was typical of neuroblastoma in that it stemmed from her adrenal gland near her kidneys. They were confident they could remove at least 95% percent of it. And they removed 100% of the monstrous thing.

St. Jude's is an amazing research hospital. "Today, St. Jude is leading the way the world understands, treats and defeats childhood cancer and other life-threatening diseases," according to their website.

"The mission of St. Jude Children's Research Hospital is to advance cures, and means of prevention, for pediatric catastrophic diseases through research and treatment." When we first went to St. Jude's Affiliate Clinic in Peoria, Illinois, the nurses and doctors were welcoming and caring. They were skilled in dealing with traumatized parents and helped us throughout the whole process.

Beyond the amazing doctors and nurses, there were social workers, financial advisors, counselors, and other resources available. Because of their mission, St. Jude's also covered any procedures or treatments done at their clinic or hospital financially. This saved us financially. Because treating a child for cancer will financially ruin you. You will stop caring about the daily struggles of life like paying bills because your child is struggling to survive. St. Jude's does its best to make sure you only have to worry about the important priorities in your life.

Things to Know

DIAGNOSIS

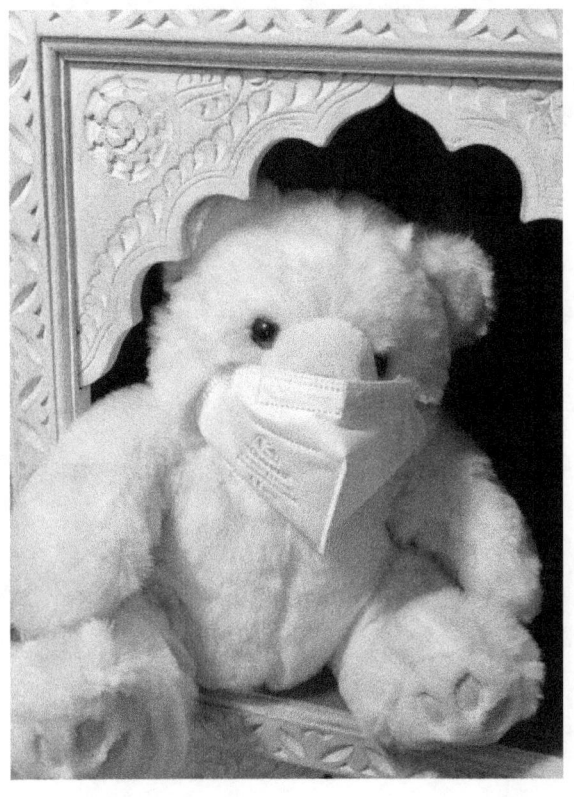

Things to Know

When she was first diagnosed, Ian and I blamed ourselves for not noticing certain details. As the doctors started to run tests, we realized it was much more complicated than we'd thought to diagnose. They not only looked at her general physical history, they did multiple urine tests to measure certain acids that were found with neuroblastoma. They took blood so many times I lost count. The first time trying to get an IV in her tiny veins was traumatic. It took over six tries, three blown veins, six nurses, and a specialty nurse called in to finally get her IV put in so they could do blood tests. They took skin samples, bone marrow biopsies, x-rays, CT scans, ultrasounds, immunochemistry tests, and MIBG scans to help determine the type and stage of cancer. The whole process made us realize we couldn't have known. Thank God we took her in for her yearly exam.

Evelyn didn't have many of the symptoms that come with neuroblastoma because it sat dormant for part of her life. I actually had extra ultrasounds when I was pregnant because there was an abnormality in the fetus near the kidneys. In hindsight, this could have been diagnosed prenatally had we paid more attention or had a doctor pushed for more answers. They were fine monitoring it and when it didn't grow prenatally, just ignoring it after birth. Some of the symptoms she didn't have included noticeable lumps in the abdomen, neck, or chest, bulging eyes, bone pain, bluish lumps under the skin, weakness or paralysis, shortness of breath, petechiae, high blood pressure, diarrhea, jerky muscle movements, uncontrolled eye movements, and swelling of legs, ankles, or feet.

Once they'd diagnosed symptoms and done tests, they staged Evelyn as Stage 4S, which meant she had tendencies that ran between intermediate and high-risk. In Stage 1, the tumor is the only threat and can be completely removed through surgery. Stage 2 has A and B sections. In 2A, the tumor is localized, but cannot be completely removed with surgery. In 2B, the tumor is localized, and can possibly be removed with surgery, although cancer cells are still found within lymph nodes around the tumor site. If the child's tumor cannot be removed and cancer has spread to the other side of the body or lymph nodes, if the child's tumor is on one side but lymph nodes are on the other side of the body, or if the child's tumor is in the middle and has spread to tissues on both sides or can't be removed, it is Stage 3. Stage 4 means that the tumor has spread to distant lymph nodes, the skin, or other parts of the body. Stage 4S, Evelyn's stage, meant that the following was mostly true: she was

Things to Know

under a year old (although not technically, she was close enough), cancer had spread to various other parts of her body, the tumor was localized and could probably be removed, and cancer cells were found in lymph nodes near the tumor site. Identifying and understanding her staging took tests and time.

How they treat neuroblastoma is based on the risk group she is put in. Low and intermediate-risk neuroblastoma have a high chance of being cured. High-risk neuroblastoma may be difficult to cure. Because of some variant factors, Evelyn was difficult to place. There was also the worry of progressive and recurrent neuroblastoma, meaning it grew resistant to treatment or came back after going away.

Treating intermediate to high risk neuroblastoma includes a number of variables and options, but the most common protocol according to the Children's Oncology Group's website, is to include four to six rounds of high-dose induction chemotherapy to reduce the growth of disease and tumors. Surgery may also be done in order to remove as much of the tumors as possible. Then generally one to two rounds of consolidation therapy, or stem cell harvest and transplant with high dose chemotherapy. This was by far the most difficult part of treatment for Evelyn physically. After these treatments, radiation is given to the primary tumor site in an attempt to avoid relapse or growth. Evelyn had a targeted kind of radiation called proton beam therapy. After this, many high risk patients must continue maintenance therapy, which includes medicines and treatments to prevent disease from growing back.

    Since neuroblastoma is such a tricky cancer to figure out, variations of these treatments can be made based on parental choices, health of the cancer child, or doctor suggestions, as well as, sadly, finances and geographical locations. There are Facebook support groups where I've read stories of children not able to get treatment because their country hasn't authorized the poisons used to combat the disease. My heart breaks for these parents and children who don't have the choices allowed in the United States. We were given the choice of one or two stem cell transplants and decided to opt out of the second one because the first one was so harsh on Evelyn. Even within our own hospital, the differing levels of care could be seen. We'd walk by rooms where parents had to work and leave children alone with nurses to care for them. We saw newborn babies who'd been abandoned because treatment became too difficult for parents to deal with. We met grandparents who were the primary caretakers during treatment because of

Things to Know

whatever circumstances. Ian and I were lucky to have each other and to have a strong support system. Too many people don't have this, causing lasting impacts like depression, divorce, and even death and suicide.

One way people can help avoid these awful events are by supporting clinical research trials. Evelyn is signed up for several, and we just report what's going on in our lives health-wise when they ask. There are trials available through various organizations that certain patients can be a part of. These trials are how new drugs come to exist. These new drugs are how we treat this disease in a more humane way. The trials generally have very specific requirements that cancer patients must meet in order to be a part of. Clinical trials can be found at Mayo Clinic in Rochester, Minnesota, Memorial Sloan Kettering Children's Hospital in New York City, the University of California in San Francisco, Seattle Children's Hospital, and other places around the world.

While we were overwhelmed with information and options that we couldn't even decipher, my daughter was overwhelmed by restrictions placed on her for health reasons. This was beyond difficult for her. You would never have guessed she was sick, watching her run and play. She loved being outside, loved our cats, loved being active, and was generally a happy-go-lucky toddler. After diagnosis, she was told she had to be masked when she was immunocompromised, isolated while she was getting treatments, tied to an IV pole and monitors, and couldn't eat cheese, her favorite food in all its forms. She wasn't allowed to see her animals unless both they and her had been cleaned and sanitized first. Don't ever take for granted the freedoms healthy children have. They can be gone in an instant when your kid becomes a cancer kid.

The first time she went under anesthesia, it was for a biopsy to determine what the doctors suspected: neuroblastoma. Neuroblastoma is one of the most common cancers found in children between the ages of 1 and 2. She had many of the symptoms suddenly, which is often the case. Reading through the list of signs, many of them are caused by the tumor pushing against nearby tissues and organs. Her stomach was swollen, she had dark circles under her eyes with fevers, and some unexplained bruising. We discovered it before her symptoms became too life-altering, thanks to her yearly check-ups. The biopsy confirmed what we knew, but was also our first experience with her being put under. She woke up fine, but her throat was scratchy for days because she'd been intubated with too large of a tube, and

Things to Know

because she'd been under for so long. We learned quickly to advocate for her comfort. There was a smaller tube, it just made the doctor's job a little bit more difficult. We asked for that tube from that point on without incident.

After the biopsy, she had tons of scans, then surgery was scheduled. Although there were spots of the cancer in her skull and around her eyes, the majority of it was just the tumor still. Surgery day was the longest time I'd ever spent in a hospital setting. We wandered and figured out where Don's Bistro was, the gift shops, the parking garage, and other various hospital areas. Getting comfortable in that setting took time and effort, but as we continue to spend time there three years later, it was something that needed to be done. As we made our way back to the waiting room, worries and fears about just this surgery, much less the rest of the treatments, nearly overwhelmed us. Having a surgeon come out and call your child's name, then walking back into the tiny room where they deliver all types of news and updates was one of the most stressful moments of my life. Thankfully, they were able to remove the entire softball-sized tumor. Unfortunately since the cancer had already spread, we were heading straight to her first round of chemotherapy.

Things to Know

TREATMENT

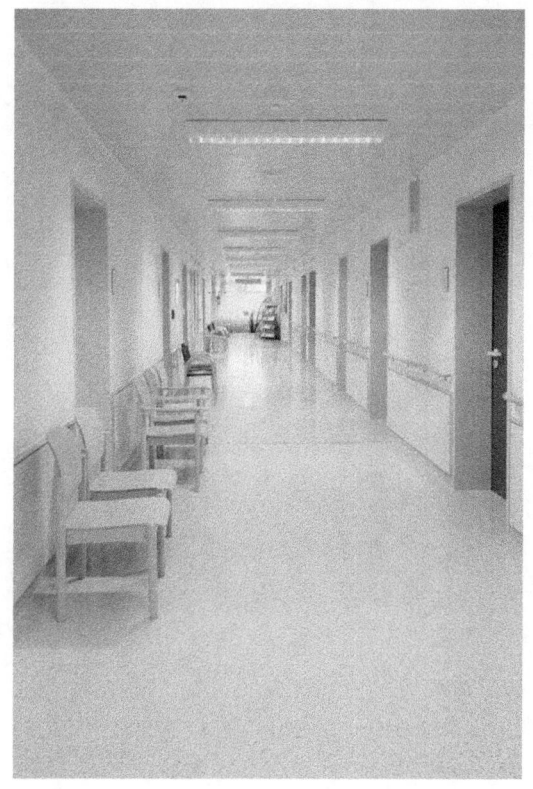

Things to Know

Before this round of chemotherapy could start, she had to have a port placed and various other things prepared. Because of her weakened condition, however, they were nervous about how invasive of a surgery it would be. They decided to put in what's called a central line, which is one of the more invasive surgeries for placing a port. Waiting for her while she was in surgery was difficult, but seeing her come back into a room, still bleeding and coding because her blood was too thin was one of many traumatic experiences we would go through in hospitals. We almost lost her for the first time that day. Ian held her, pressing on her chest wound where the port was to stop the bleeding. They were transfusing blood directly into her while trying to contain the damage. Her oxygen levels bottomed out and people were called in for emergency treatment. It's amazing what the mind can take and hide away in order to be able to cope and move forward from traumatic experiences.

Our first round of chemotherapy included two days of preparing, five days of treatment, and one to two days of recovery. Preparing meant blood and urine tests to make sure she was healthy enough for her body to receive the toxins in the chemotherapy drugs. This is a common part of treatment.

She was a trooper and handled things far better than I did. I let her run the hallways outside of our hospital room, chasing her with her IV so she didn't pull out her fluids or medicine. It was stressful and worrisome, and some of the nurses and patients looked at us like we were crazy. But she needed to run and I needed to let her. Making sure she had everything she needed to be happy and comfortable became a priority in my life, nearly an obsession. It's an urge I have to fight today, even though we are years out of treatment.

The first time we went home after diagnosis, we ended up back in the hospital in under twenty-four hours. She'd spiked a low-grade fever, but that could be deadly to a cancer kid. Going home had been the scariest, bravest thing we'd done. We were so overwhelmed by everything we'd be taking care of, but so ready to be home. Or so we thought. One of the main things the nurses and doctors reiterated to us was how dangerous a fever could be. We knew as we drove home her temperature was rising, but the hope of getting home made us continue to monitor it until it was too high to deny we needed to head back. Fevers and reactions would haunt us throughout her treatment, like many other cancer patients. Fevers equal fear is still a reaction I have to fight to this day.

Things to Know

We learned the hard way how to pack quickly. In the middle of the night, after being gone for nearly three weeks, we had to throw things into overnight bags, including Penny's things, and make a trip back to the hospital. After that trip, we realized having an emergency bag packed was crucial. We included the obvious like pajamas and toiletries, but also the not-so-obvious ones like things to keep them distracted. Evelyn loved movies and she called our phones "Troll's phone" because she used to watch Trolls the movie over and over again on them. We brought soft and small toys, and used our wagon that we'd purchased for Penny's sporting events to haul things in and out of the hospital. Family and friends send cards and posters and signs and decorations to help cheer us up, so we used those to decorate her room. Many of the nurses complimented us on the effort we put in.

Nurses are the glue that holds hospitals and families together. When we called St. Jude's to tell them we were coming in hot with a fever, they got a room ready for us and welcomed us with caring, open arms. Their ward was full, but they found space. We ended up with a larger corner room since Penny came with us. It was one of the only overnight trips she took to the hospital with us during treatment.

We made the decision to keep her relatively distant during actual treatment. We learned that every family deals with this differently, choosing the best strategy for their family dynamics and needs. We were lucky to have an amazing support system at home that allowed us to provide a modicum of normality to our other child. She wasn't forced to spend nights in a Ronald McDonald house, but got to sleep in her own bed, with her pets and family around.

Many families who don't have support systems must leave their homes and live temporarily in Ronald McDonald houses. This is an amazing organization, and again, I know there are several similar organizations and resources around the world, but it doesn't take the place of being at home. We did make use of these resources later in her treatment, however, learning that there are valid reasons for these resources to be there. During her radiation treatment, Evelyn and Ian stayed up in the Chicago suburbs three and a half hours from our house. Ronald McDonald House Charities allowed them to have a home away from home while Penny and I did the weekly role of school and work, then visited on the weekends. Ronald McDonald House Charities "believes when families are together, they cope better. [They] believe no family should have to deal with their child's medical crisis alone."

RHMC not only offered us a chance to be together during treatment, it offered us a chance to participate in a community that understood what we were going through. Evelyn made friends with two little girls around her age that were also staying there. Heartbreakingly, one of the little girls passed away two years after we were done with treatment. They were still fighting her battle. One of the scariest parts of treatment is the fact that it can cause other diseases and complications. This is what happened to her. The other little girl is doing well and recently had clear scans. The Ronald McDonald House Charity became a common link that helped us cope with and make the best of a trying time in our lives.

We were able to see Penny during our two week breaks in between chemotherapy treatments. We tried to live life normally, taking her to as many practices and games as we could make. I attempted to work for the first part of treatment, but soon realized I needed time off to focus on family. After choosing Penny's soccer tournament over a volleyball match I was supposed to coach, I resigned my volleyball coaching position and took leave from my teaching position. My husband, Ian, took time off as well. We were ironically lucky in the timing of it, as we were both schoolteachers. We had to learn to look for luck in every situation. She was diagnosed right at the end of the school year, which meant we had the summer to deal with the initial shock and transition of living life with a cancer kid.

Another thing that we clung to for hope was Evelyn's vitality and love of life. Whenever we said we were heading to Peoria, where her treatments were, she got excited because the clinic had a giant playroom. Take advantage of every opportunity you have to let your child play. She loved the giant dollhouse, and the train set. Her favorite part was the fish tank and she loved to play with the little kitchen set. The social worker was always friendly and made the best of the shittiest situations.

One of the shittiest moments was when she started losing her hair. She didn't start losing her hair until the 2nd round of chemotherapy. I told myself over and over that it was not a big deal, but she had been born with a full head of thick, black hair. Watching it fall out because of the poisons we were forced to use to kill her cancer was traumatizing for me and my husband. I cannot think about it to this day without crying. The first time I brushed through her hair and a chunk came out, reality hit like a hammer. We held

Things to Know

onto those wispy, dark strands. Still have them in a ziploc baggie stored away with our other treatment memories/nightmares. Deciding how to talk about treatment with your cancer kid is a personal and individualized choice parents must make. Evelyn was young enough that she doesn't remember everything, thank God. But she remembers just enough for it to make life confusing and challenging every now and then. We've discussed several different ways of approaching it, and still haven't decided on a course of action. We answer questions honestly as she has them, but don't think she's ready to actually comprehend the battle she fought and the tragedy she survived.

Evelyn survived four rounds of chemotherapy, two rounds of immunotherapy, spread out throughout the next year, each round lasting about a week. Then we'd take a two or three week break, depending on how harsh the chemotherapy had been and how quickly Evelyn recovered. The amount of chemistry and biology we learned throughout the process was mind-blowing. We also learned anatomy and physiology, medical jargon, hospital hierarchy, and our own limits. I don't remember much of it, as it was a dark time period, but learning about her white blood cell counts, and vanillylmandelic acid tests, and

Broviac Hickman ports, and PICC lines, and so many other horrible things, made me realize that ignorance is actually bliss.

When she first started chemotherapy, then immunotherapy, our only priority was her survival. We didn't know the difference between chemotherapy and immunotherapy, but we quickly learned. Chemotherapy attacks the cancer cells using toxins and drugs. It's effects are harsh and often long-term, causing other types of cancer and disability. Immunotherapy uses the body's immune system to attack cancer cells. Although just as harsh in some side effects, this has less chance of causing other diseases. Some cancers require a combination of both, such as Evelyn's.

As we got into a routine that included days in the hospital in isolation, we went from living and enjoying life fully as a family, to struggling in survival mode. We learned about entertaining a sick toddler, sitting through hours in a lumpy hospital chair, enduring the crying in pain, suffering through holding her down to administer medicines, and having warnings for medicines read to us because they're so dangerous. Learning to shower when she was asleep or drugged enough to be sleeping. Figuring out when to ask the nurses for a coffee run.

Things to Know

Understanding the beeps and lights and alarms that constantly surround you while you're trying to function and keep life normal.

Things to Know

RESOURCES

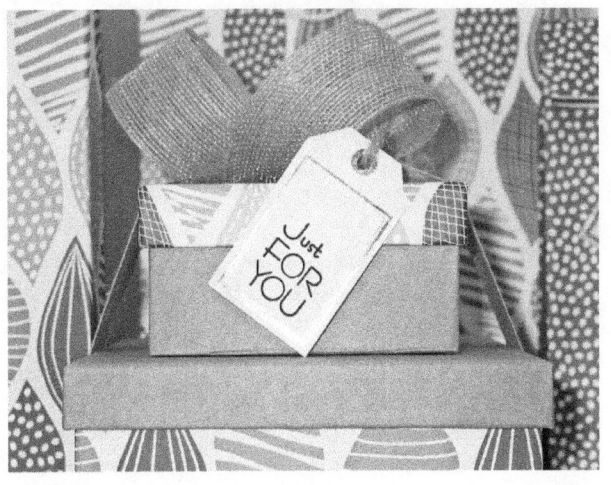

Things to Know

Bills will come, whether or not you're ready to pay them. They will still come while your child is fighting for her life. There will still be due dates and insurance issues. The fight to get things paid for was almost too much for us. Use your FMLA and sick bank days and any other resources your employer can afford to give you. Losing pay from being gone, while trying to pay for the reason you're gone is a horrible cycle that can tear apart families and cause many to not get the treatment options they should.

I was fortunate enough to have some great friends put together fundraisers for us. We wouldn't have made it out with as little debt as we did if they hadn't organized and publicized and worked to make things happen. Let your friends help. Mine organized a volleyball tournament with a raffle and other donation activities. The proceeds went toward her treatment and transportation costs back and forth from Peoria St. Jude. Ian's school district collected gift cards and donated sick days to his sick bank. My school district did multiple fundraisers and sent cards and uplifting messages. Without our support systems, we would never be back to living the life we wanted for our girls.

While Evelyn was lucky enough to win her battle against cancer, so many childhood warriors are not.

Sadly, it's often complications from the treatment that ends up taking their life. Their bodies become so weak they cannot handle the chemotherapy. Or organs start to shut down and doctors can't take action because the normal surgery would kill the cancer kid. Or they are in so much pain, multiple medicines are given and mistakes can be made. This is what almost happened to Evelyn during her stem cell transplant. She coded and stopped breathing while we were holding her after having medicine administered by a nurse who was new to us. We nearly lost her again that day, but thanks to the team of doctors and nurses, disaster was averted and we still have her with us.

Many charities are formed from the tragedies of other families. A family local to us had lost their little boy to complications from cancer treatment around the same time we were going through treatment. They started the Brantley Francis Foundation in honor of him and to help other cancer kids get through treatment. Their fundraisers generally go toward childhood cancer research organizations or their BFF bags. The BFF bags include toys and educational items for children going through treatment. I honestly don't know how his parents get up each day, but they do and they do amazing things for other people.

Things to Know

They're part of the reason I was inspired to start writing this. I need to face my trauma in order to be able to help others.

Another charity is Jessie Raes Foundation, which was actually created by a young cancer patient who wanted to make a difference. Jessie was a twelve-year-old girl who fought cancer for a little over a year before gaining her angel wings. She created "Joy Jars," which are jars full of entertaining goodies for cancer kids. She also coined the term "NEGU," or Never Ever Give Up, to inspire cancer patients and families to continue to fight. Not only for their lives, but for funding and age-appropriate research.

While globally there was over 167 billion dollars spent on cancer research, only around 4% of that, or about 6.6 billion dollars go toward childhood cancer research. This is flabbergasting considering childhood cancer is the number one cause of death by disease among children. The article entitled "Gap between pediatric and adult approvals of molecular targeted drugs," reported that in the United States, Europe, and Japan "a total of 103 drugs were approved for adult patients in at least one of the three regions whereas only 10 drugs were approved for pediatric patients." Children are not mini-adults and have physical differences that can be life-threatening or saving, depending on the treatment. We need to come up with more options and treatment plans for saving these children. The ones we were offered were so toxic, you had to decide whether your priority was to survive the disease or the treatment for the disease.

The Facebook Community was another resource that was extremely supportive. Although sometimes the information and stories from the groups broke your heart, many times they offered invaluable information about treatment options, how to advocate for your child, or what people regretted. Seeing parents with the same doubts helped us be strong when we needed to be. It also allowed us to seek help when we needed to. Although we are not the most interactive in the groups, they have inspired me to start facing my trauma by writing this book. I want to help other people, and in order to do that without breaking down and crying constantly, I need to start dealing with how her treatment made me feel.

Every time we came home, there was a sense of relief, but also fear and worry. I cannot reiterate the importance of accepting and even asking for help during this process. If my parents and in-laws, aunts and uncles, cousins and friends hadn't taken care of our house, pets, food, and homecoming, it would have been even more of a nightmare than it was. We were

Things to Know

worried about her comfort and sanitizing everything and not hurting her port. Often after treatment, she was nauseous, weak, and irritable. She wanted to fit in as much play and activity as she could. Sleeping only happened when she'd worn herself into the ground running around. Eating was a challenge because her tastebuds were changing due to chemotherapy and immunotherapy treatments.

Things to Know

MORE TREATMENT

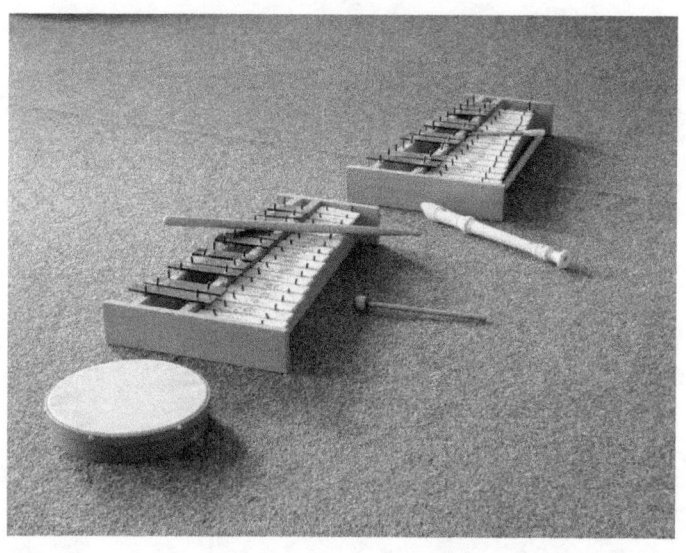

Things to Know

Home wasn't always the safe place we hoped it would be for her either. We still had to flush her port so that it continued to function between treatments. When we went home in between in-patient rounds, there were also certain medicines we had to give. Some were oral, which was a challenge with a toddler, even one not on cancer treatments. Some of the oral meds had side effects. Others were shots we had to give to build up certain antibodies in her body to help deal with the side effects of treatment. It took both my husband and myself to hold her down most times. Some days we even had Penny help by holding the Ipad or phone to distract her. I wonder what effect this experience had on their relationship, but we had to do what we had to do to survive.

Throughout chemotherapy and immunotherapy, Ian and I had rotated as often as we could, with one of us doing in-patient treatment while the other stayed with Penny. After that part of treatment, she started preparing for a stem cell harvest and transplant. Harvest and transplant are where the rebuilding of her disease-free immune system begins. Her schedule was actually changed around to have immunotherapy first because scans came back that her disease wasn't responding as well to chemotherapy as they'd hoped. Then Evelyn went through one harvest and transplant, although some patients require two transplants if their disease was more prominent or aggressive. This part of treatment is where her injections were required the most. Her body had to create a certain number of stem cells to be harvested. The stem cell harvest ended up being a weekend-long nightmare. The first day, her numbers weren't where they needed to be, which meant we made the trip to Chicago for nothing. The next day, the machine kept malfunctioning. This not only meant keeping her sedated longer than normal, which has a whole host of side effects, but also meant getting rid of some of her precious stem cells. To make matters worse, her harvest started on a Friday, so pushing it back meant we were spending the weekend in the hospital, rather than just a couple days. I spent three days on a couch next to her hospital bed, unable to hold her or move her, waiting on tenterhooks for her to flinch or cry out during the actual harvest. We did what we do best and survived so that she could recover enough in order to start the next process.

The stem cell transplant was the scariest in my mind. It's scariest for a couple of reasons. First because the side effects are so harsh they can literally kill you. Secondly because it can be unsuccessful. If the stem cells don't engraft, all of that suffering and

Things to Know

risk is for nothing. We'd known another local family who lost their teenage-aged son during the time of Evelyn's treatment. He was a soccer player who Ian had coached until he was too sick to play anymore. He'd undergone chemotherapy and stem cell transplant, but had used a donor's stem cells instead of his own. When the transplant had failed, our hearts had been broken. He eventually passed away from the side effects that his weakened body could no longer handle. We went into transplant with his story fresh in our minds and hearts. Looking back on Facebook posts from that time, I can't stop the tears. "Yesterday was easy but long...drive to Chicago, have some blood work done, sign some consent forms, then drive home. However, I am not sure Ian and I are ready to live up there the next few months during stem cell transplant. We are not ready to miss Penny for weeks at a time. We are not ready to watch Evelyn get sick and sad and tired. We have been planning this procedure for months (nearly 6 months now) but we are not really ready. Scans came back that show her disease is stable, but it is still in her skull and several other spots. They can't tell without more scans if they are dead spots or live spots of cancer cells. Going to transplant is somewhat risky because she isn't completely clear of the disease. But it's what our doctors are recommending. Please pray that we can be ready in time for next week, that our doctors are thinking of Evelyn as more than just a case study number, and that Penny can adjust to this lifestyle change for the next few months. #fucancer #curechildhoodcancer #sheisapersontoo #bigsisterlove."

Many patients receive treatment in multiple locations, but being in a different city and new hospital that we were unfamiliar with didn't help our anxiety at all. Although the playroom was above and beyond what she was used to, we were still nervous about our decision to start transplant. When one of our first interactions included a nurse nearly overdosing Evelyn on pain medications, we were even more fearful we'd made a mistake with her treatment plan. After food service left the outside door open three different times, allowing contaminants into the isolated, air-filtered room, we'd had enough and started advocating aggressively for her safety. Once we made it clear we knew what we were doing and were not afraid to speak up for our child, the treatment got better.

Learning to communicate effectively with doctors, nurses, and different scheduling departments takes practice in itself. At the start of the transplant, Evelyn didn't pass some baseline tests for her kidneys and bowel functions, which meant the transplant got pushed back. Then, after I head home and Ian stays in Chicago, there's a surgery scheduled. Nothing major, but something I would have stayed for.

Evelyn bullied her way through transplant with the same gusto she'd attacked the rest of her treatment plan. Her energy was through the roof compared to other children, making her confinement in a twelve-by-twelve foot isolation room one of the most burdensome tasks for Ian and me. Keeping her entertained took an army. She had several harsh reactions to the transplant, making it hard for her to eat and stay hydrated. She worked with physical therapists to avoid muscle atrophy since she spent most of her day hooked up to IV's and monitors in a hospital bed. Musical therapists came in, social workers came in, so many specialists and doctors I couldn't even tell you her primary doctor's name from that time.

After her stem cell transplant was considered an official success based on a number of tests, she and Ian stayed in a Ronald McDonald House for a week, then Penny and I joined them for the weekend. Looking back on that time from Team Evelyn's Facebook page, "We had a wonderful weekend together as a whole family. It was difficult to send Penny back to school while we stay for appointments Monday and Tuesday this week. Just when I was starting to get depressed about it, I hopped on Facebook and got a reality check. Please pray for the Francis family of Geneseo who lost their three year old son, Brantley, today after a lifetime battle with health issues. My heart is breaking for them and once again for this small community that I call home. I will always remember, even at our darkest times, there are those who have it darker. When we feel strong, there are those who are stronger. And during our weakest, most vulnerable times, we can still help others. #TeamBrantley #TrevStrong #Livelikeapenguin #TeamEvelyn." I learned that spreading this message is more important than hiding from my trauma.

    The next portion of her treatment plan was radiation. She would spend a month in a Ronald McDonald House in Chicago. Ian had taken off work and I would stay with Penny for the month. It seemed like years. Each day, they would go to the treatment center and receive radiation treatment. She would put on her mask to sleep in and get sent into this big white machine where they pumped a specialized proton beam therapy through her original cancer sites. This is to help prevent the cancer from coming back, but is more targeted so there are less likely to be secondary cancers. Her daily treatment times were short, but it was wearing on her body. The Ronald McDonald House allowed Ian and her to recover in privacy. Her appetite during this time dipped so low that we had to use nutritional supplements and an NG tube. Her immunity was also extremely low, meaning she wore a mask everywhere and visitors were strictly monitored. I came up on the weekends, or if Ian needed a break, he came home on the weekends. We never wanted to be far from medical help, however, so we tried to keep her centrally located. She maintained her hilarious personality, loving to make people laugh and be silly.

We were finally together as a family again over Christmas of 2017. Welcoming them home felt amazing, but scary at the same time. There was a sense of relief, followed quickly by panic. What did we do now that we didn't need to live in survival mode anymore? Sure there were still things we had to monitor and do. Part of her post-treatment plan included accutane, an extremely strong medication usually used to prevent horrible acne. The chemicals in the drug apparently also attack cancer cells, which is amazing news. However, the side effects of the drug are quite harsh. It's a slippery little pill that's basically poison inside. If touched, it can actually cause burns and other cancerous side effects.

Scans are the scariest, yet most reassuring part of treatment. After transplant, hers still unfortunately showed signs of disease in her skull. This meant continuing with more immunotherapy. Immunotherapy side effects include all of the normal, as well as incredible neuropathic pain. She took drugs to help build up her tolerance to the treatment, but she hated taking them. We had to get creative with it, and eventually just straight forceful about it. We did a round after not having her take it faithfully and her pain was off the charts.

We did six rounds of immunotherapy post-radiation before she had scans to hopefully be declared NED, or no evidence of disease. Each round of immunotherapy was its own different kind of hell, from bacterial infections that meant her central line port had to be removed and replaced, to rashes and infections, to fevers that wouldn't break, to poor pain management despite our suggestions and wishes. Unfortunately her scans afterwards showed lit up spots that were inconclusive. This didn't mean more treatment but it did mean more monitoring.

After her treatment was finished, we started planning her Make-A-Wish trip. She decided on

Things to Know

Disneyworld and it was amazing. In December of 2019, we were spoiled from the start. A limo picked us up and took us to the airport. We were lucky enough to be staying at the Give Kids the World Village, where meals and entertainment were provided in a setting with accessible medical services. It was a magical trip and we honestly probably could have spent the whole week in the pool at the Village. However, our itinerary was busy, including most of the Disney parks that were age appropriate. The girls' favorite was Animal Kingdom. We also attended a Medieval Times Dinner and tried indoor skydiving. Even Evelyn! It was a once-in-a-lifetime trip that had us worn out by the time we got home. Good thing Make-A-Wish provided a limo driver to and from the airport.

Things to Know

OUR LIFE CURRENTLY

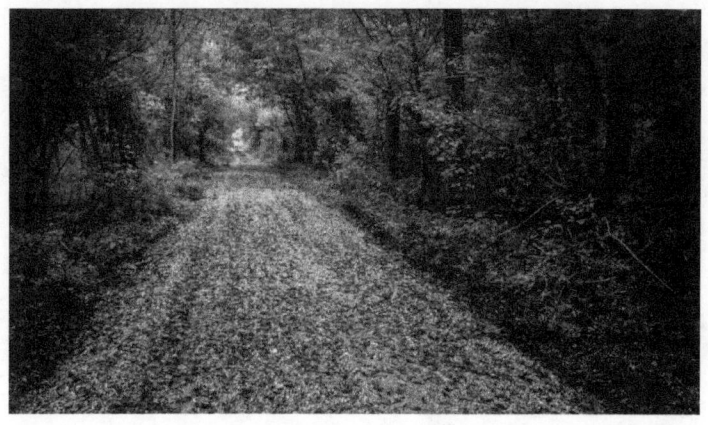

Things to Know

The end of treatment doesn't mean the end of doctor and hospital visits. It means we got to stretch them out with more time in between. This was a blessing and a curse. More time in between meant feeling like life was getting back to normal. It also meant worrying and stressing about the little aches and pains that she had in between scan times. At first, it was a clinic check-up every couple weeks. Scans were three months apart, then they progressed to six months, then nine months. Now we are yearly, and will eventually be stretched out even farther apart.

So just when we thought life was about to return to normal, the COVID pandemic hit. It made me realize everyone has a different normal. Our normal included masks before they were the thing. It also included extreme sanitization to the point of having fancy hand sanitizers installed in our home. So most of the precautions we were taking weren't unusual for us. I realized other people did not feel the same way when the controversy over masks began. My feelings on that could fill a whole different book.

Now we're dealing with a whole host of challenges. The most obvious include monitoring side effects from her treatment. Her growth is a focus of ours. And she often complains of her temperature being too hot or too cold. One of the chemotherapy treatments warned of growth limitations and early menopause, so we're afraid she may experience that. She also complains of leg growth, which in our mind could be growing pains, could be cancerous tumors. And as she's started Kindergarten in 2021, we are noticing limitations and learning challenges that may or may not be related to treatment. My husband is severely ADHD and dyslexic, so it's difficult to say if her struggles are genetic, or brought on from treatment.

Mentally and emotionally, dealing with cancer has made Evelyn one of the toughest children we know. And as teachers, we know a lot of children. Despite this, we're dealing with the fall-out of making the world all about her and using prizes for pain tolerance. We have a ton of toys because she feels like she always needs gifts because it was a part of her life. She got a shot, then she'd get a gift. She had blood drawn, she earned a prize. It just became a habit. And as a parent, it was a tough habit to get away from. Now our house is filled with toys and trinkets. We're working on the idea of giving things away and helping those less fortunate than us, but it fights against her nature of getting rewarded for tasks.

This frustrates Penelope constantly. Penny isn't a child who needs a lot of things. The state of our house

Things to Know

with all of the toys often stresses her out. Seeing her sister treated differently, and knowing that she sometimes gets away with selfish/spoiled behavior also breeds some resentment. She is so understanding about what her sister went through and how it affects her, but she also feels left out sometimes. Be careful not to isolate the cancer kid's siblings in an effort to protect them. Sometimes I worry that's what we did with Penny, and we're doing our best to make sure we don't continue to make her feel that way.

Ian and I also dealt with the consequences of having a cancer child. Our emotional state is much more fragile. Although we've lived through hell and made it, that feeling of must-survive haunts us, causing stress. This stress usually causes us to lash out at each other. Although we both realize it's happening and know why, it doesn't make dealing with it any easier. We've also dealt with a loss of friends and the lack of drive to even have a social life. Sleep is a hit-or-miss experience in our house, as during treatment, Evelyn always had one of us in her room with her. She has to have one of us with her to fall asleep, which has definitely caused distance between Ian and I.

The role of religion and faith throughout all of this will obviously depend on the individuals involved.

Initially, I couldn't figure out why God, or whoever, would do this to us. Was it some kind of test? A punishment of some sort? Why would this happen? But even as I questioned it, I knew she would beat it. I never doubted for a minute that she would come out on top. There's the faith I had. The one that I kept. My faith in her and in science. My faith in the idea that she was meant for something bigger, something far more grandiose than dying from cancer or cancer treatments. My faith that my little girl is going to change the world for the better was what allowed me to hang on at times. Some families will turn to their home church. Others will utilize the hospital chapel, while others will turn completely away from any kind of organized faith. I will never be able to judge what another parent does to survive their child's treatment.

Another mother of a cancer kid expressed it perfectly:

Imagine…

Imagine being told your child is seriously ill.

Imagine crying until you think there's nothing left.

Imagine feeling like you've been punched in the stomach and wandering the corridors, as if your life was on pause for days on end, weeks, months, not able to comprehend what is happening.

Things to Know

Imagine signing a consent form knowing that death is a possibility.

Imagine having to hand over your child to surgeons over and over for endless hours and waiting…

Imagine having to watch as your once active child isn't even able to open their eyes for a week.

Imagine your child covered in wires with a machine breathing for them.

Imagine seeing your child resuscitated and been so close to leaving you.

Imagine the terror…

Imagine the pain of having to leave your baby in the care of strangers and not be able to sleep by their side.

Imagine standing by as your baby's body is pumped full of medication.

Imagine holding your baby down countless times while someone sticks needles in them while they scream.

Imagine the guilt…

Imagine you keep being told the percentage chances that your child might survive or leave you.

Imagine holding back the tears when your other children are carried away from you screaming "mummy" not understanding why you won't come home.

Imagine not being able to leave the house for fear of infection.

Imagine not being able to make any plans apart from hospital visits.

Imagine being stuck in isolation and not seeing anything but four walls for days on end.

Imagine learning a whole new vocabulary of words which is all you talk about anymore.

Imagine good friends being too uncomfortable to see you or speak to you anymore.

Imagine the loneliness…

Imagine perfect strangers passing comment about your daughter/son.

But with the emptiness…

Imagine the kindness of strangers who don't know you.

Imagine the incredible support from people you've never met but know how it feels.

Imagine how special each cuddle is that you feel the need to memorize it.

Imagine the magic of each smile knowing that this smile was lost for weeks and now it's back.

Imagine how fragile and precious life feels.

Things to Know

Imagine having to hold your child while they struggle to breathe.

Imagine holding your child tight while struggling not to sob uncontrollably while they take their last breath in your arms and you can't help them.

Imagine NEVER hearing or seeing your child again.

Imagine...Don't pity. Don't sympathize. Just spread awareness and just imagine, because it could happen to anyone.

So besides donating money, what are some ways you can support local cancer families? Offer to drive them to and from the hospital. Although this may take some coordination and timing, it can also save money, energy, and time. Another way to help is to give local or hospital coffee shop gift cards, gas cards, or other gift cards. You can always pick a common chore and take care of it for the family. One woman's mother-in-law hired a weekly housekeeper to take the stress off. Freezer meals are also always appreciated. Gifts and presents or activities for siblings can also help out. DVDs or streaming subscriptions are excellent gifts to keep isolated families entertained. You could also offer to take care of their pets or plants if applicable. All of these were things people did or helped get done for us throughout treatment. Without that support, going back to a regular life would have taken us much longer. Although it's important for research to be funded, it's also important for these families to survive comfortably in the darkest times of their lives. If you know a parent whose child has been affected by cancer, don't be afraid to reach out.

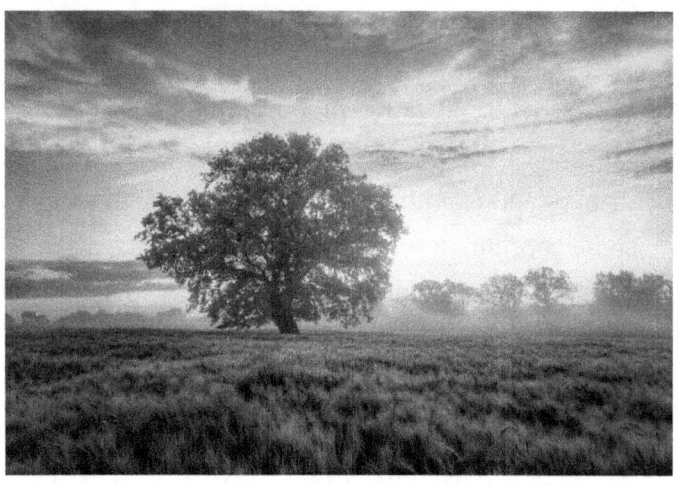

Things to Know

OTHER HELPFUL RESOURCES

St. Jude's Children's Research Hospital -
www.stjude.org

Memorial Sloan-Kettering Cancer Center -
www.mskcc.org

Young Lives vs. Cancer -
https://www.younglivesvscancer.org.uk/

READ OTHER 50 THINGS TO KNOW BOOKS

50 Things to Know About Coping With Stress: By A Mental Health Specialist by Kimberly L. Brownridge

50 Things to Know About Being a Zookeeper: Life of a Zookeeper by Stephanie Fowlie

50 Things to Know About Becoming a Doctor: The Journey from Medical School of the Medical Profession by Tong Liu MD

50 Things to Know About Knitting: Knit, Purl, Tricks & Shortcuts by Christina Fanelli

50 Things to Know

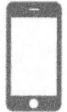

Stay up to date with new releases on Amazon:
https://amzn.to/2VPNGr7

CZYKPublishing.com

50 Things to Know

We'd love to hear what you think about our content! Please leave your honest review of this book on Amazon and Goodreads. We appreciate your positive and constructive feedback. Thank you.

www.ingramcontent.com/pod-product-compliance
Lightning Source LLC
Chambersburg PA
CBHW070118230526
45472CB00004B/1317